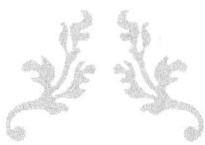

The Ultimate Guide To Getting Off Prescription Medications

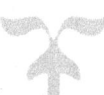

Banji Awosika

PREFACE

My father and every one of his siblings had hypertension. At the time I was deciding my career path, he had lost a SIBLING due to complications of hypertension. I had always known I wanted to help people who had the same health issues as my dad. Due to my academic quests, he saw the potential for me to become a doctor. After a few years in medical school, I left for a year to improve my financial situation. Amongst my many jobs was working as a cab driver in London, UK. I actually fell in love with medicine after I had left it for a while. So I finally came to the realization that this was what I was actually called to do.

Taking care and servicing the needs people have, educating people, and showing them how to get healthier, lessening and eventually eliminating the need for medication. Taking care and servicing the needs that people have, as well as hearing from the families of the patients that I am taking care of are amongst the most rewarding aspects that I experience as a physician. Seeing the impact on their lives is also very rewarding. When the mother of a patient comes back and tells me they lost ten pounds and that they are off medications themselves; that blesses the socks off of me. The whole idea is to create ambassadors of this message, from the patients to the staff that work with me as well as the families of the patients. That's when I can really make a difference.

This book is for daily prescription medication users, who want to know how to and who want to get off these medications and have no idea where to start. Let's get started.

Banji Awosika 21-Sep-2016

TABLE OF CONTENTS

PREFACE ii

TABLE OF CONTENTS iii

CHAPTER ONE

HOW CAN I GET OFF PRESCRIPTION MEDICATIONS 1

CHAPTER TWO

WHY DOES MY PHYSICIAN NOT GET ME OFF MEDS 6

CHAPTER THREE

HOW CAN I LOSE WEIGHT AND KEEP IT OFF? 9

CHAPTER FOUR

WHAT CAN I EAT FOR BREAKFAST? 13

CHAPTER FIVE

WHICH IS WORSE FOR ME, SIMPLE CARBS OR FATTY FOODS? 17

CHAPTER SIX

IS EATING FISH HEALTHY? 20

CHAPTER SEVEN

HOW MUCH SLEEP DO I REALLY NEED PER NIGHT? 23

THE ENDING CHAPTER

CHAPTER ONE

HOW CAN I GET OFF PRESCRIPTION MEDICATIONS

More veggies per day

In vegetables you have much more fiber and as a result of the increased fiber content there is less calorie content in the food in question. This also leads to a decrease in the transit time through the gut and as a result of this, less calories are absorbed into the blood from the gut. There is also an increase in the PH of the blood, that is, the blood becomes more alkaline. And as a result of a more alkaline blood there is less calcium leaching from the bone with consequently less of an incidence of osteoporosis and generalized increase in bone health.

Now the phytochemicals, which are chemicals that you find in plants, generally result in a decrease in incidence and prevalence of many of the chronic diseases that plague our society today. There are numerous phytochemicals, many of which have been described, but many more which have not yet been described and are yet to be found. These phytochemicals act as potent antioxidants which function to decrease chronic inflammation in our systems.

Daily fruits

Ideally, there should be fruits consumed before every meal. Fruits also are choker full of antioxidants and phytochemicals which as noted above, have an awesome affect on inflammatory processes that go on in the body, affecting various processes in the body to the body's detriment. The best kind of fruits to actually consume are berries. That is any kind of berries - strawberries, blueberries, blackberries, raspberries - as these have the most number-- highest concentration of antioxidants.

Fruits in general are high in fiber and although there is a high sugar content, the way this is packaged it has no negative effects in our body as various studies have shown. A particular study that was done to demonstrate the effects of over consuming fruits on a daily basis resulted in one major side effect which was having quite a number of bulky stools per day - a problem many people would give anything to have.

Legumes

Legumes refer to beans, lentils, chickpeas, split peas, hummus and these have a very interesting role in our diet, as they actually behave like fiber. They are actually very filling and the specific starch found in legumes called amylose actually functions effectively as fiber.

Soybeans have been used to make creative alternatives to our typical animal proteins that are consumed and in moderation actually provide a nice alternative to the typical animal proteins that are consumed.

So Although beans contain some starch, that is, legumes generally contain starch, the type of starch that make up a large part of the starch bank in beans functions as fiber resulting in all the benefits that are found in fiber. Also there is a very high protein content in beans, and this also deters the absorption of glucose into the blood from the gut. The regular absorption of glucose is also decreased by the high amylose to amylopectin ratio in beans. Generally, there is about three to nine grams of both soluble and insoluble fiber per half cup of beans. They have a very low fat content, less than 3% of total caloric value. They are also very high in iron, zinc, folates, magnesium, omega-three fatty acids, and antioxidants. There are also phytates and phenolic compounds in beans, and these function as amylase inhibitors similar to the role metformin has in increasing insulin sensitivity in patients that have diabetes.

Exercise

Exercise leads in general to better eating habits and the consequent weight loss leads to a decreased incidence in chronic disease. Exercise has many benefits and these include:

- Increasing energy consumption
- Improved cardiovascular function improved digestion
- Improved sleep hygiene
- Improved muscle and skin tone

As this involves motion, anything that involves a change in motion results in a change in emotion as well. Exercise results in the release of certain feel-good hormones that have a tendency to make us feel good and takes us on a natural high, which the body tends to crave. Unfortunately, with the high comes a low. And a withdrawal syndrome can ensue until another source is tapped into to again achieve this much sought-after high.

Looking for appropriate sources of this high is the ideal situation. Various things can create the appropriate source for a high. These include:

- Good relationship
- Rest
- Anything you're passionate about
- Sweet or savory food.

The last two sources mentioned may be appropriate or not based on frequency and quantity. So in the right frequency and quantity, these are appropriate sources of the feel-good hormone.

Another advantage of exercise is improved bone health, as weight bearing improves the health of bones and incidentally, lack of weight bearing actually increases osteoporosis and results in worsening bone health.

Animal protein

This forms the biggest portal of fat intake into our system. In animal protein there is much more saturated fat than unsaturated fat, as well as cholesterol and both retard the loss of cholesterol in the stool, increasing the cholesterol load in the body. Of course with fat there is no fiber content with all the negative effects of low fiber content of food eaten. There is an increase in the transit time as a result of the fat content of animal proteins. An increase in absorption of calories from the gut into the blood is results from this increased transit time.

There is an increased risk of chronic diseases and its progression as a result of the fatty content of animal proteins.

Smaller portions of complex carbs

Ideally our plates should not be more than one quarter as regards to the portion of carbs. One quarter of the plate should be carbs while the remaining three quarters are a mixture of veggies, fruits, and beans. Amount of carbohydrates consumed should not be more than the amount of energy that would be consumed by exercise that day. Complex carbs when consumed have a beneficial depot effect that results in a blunting of the insulin spike. This is very important in decreasing the amount of fat stored especially centrally as a result of increased circulating insulin.

Essentially hyperinsulinemia can result from hyperglycemia in obese individuals and actually result in overeating and because of the inefficient uptake of glucose by cells in these individuals, there's a conversion of this into fat. So with the flat profile of the insulin spike, the cells stay in starvation mode, which results in breakdown of fat and protein for energy if there is an absolute absence of insulin, which is also a negative situation, so having enough insulin to prevent both extremes is the ideal situation.

Minerals and Vitamin

The right minerals and vitamin intake is also very important but there should be an avoidance of salty food, especially in patients that have a little bit of blood pressure and fluid retention. Many individuals are salt sensitive. There are however certain individuals who need salt for survival in which case there is no evidence of high blood pressure or fluid retention. In this subset of individuals, without adequate salt intake, they generally have increased mortality. Majority of individuals don't have high blood pressure or fluid retention and do okay whether they have salt in their diet or not.

One out of three individuals over the age of 20 today have elevated blood pressure. Almost half of these individuals have elevated blood pressure that is not adequately treated. These individuals definitely benefit from a decrease in salt intake. I actually tell my patients to stop adding salt to their food and to look at the label and avoid consuming any product that has more than 150 milligrams per serving of sodium.

Many minerals are important in terms of quantity taken, especially with a plant-based diet. An important one I will mention here is iodine, which tends to be decreased because of certain chemicals found in a plant-based diet that are goitrogenic - goiter producing. This is especially the case when the individual is not adding salt to food which tends to be a very common source of iodine these days. Alternative sources of iodine intake is then recommended.

Other vitamins that need to be supplemented with a plant-based diet include vitamin D and vitamin B12. Vitamin D tends to come more from fortified dairy and eggs, fish which have their own issues, as well as the sun. Unfortunately, the same source, that is the sun, is also responsible for many skin cancers, so a fine balance has to be reached in amount of sun exposure. I generally recommend a vitamin D supplement for most of my patients. Especially if the levels checked demonstrate a vitamin D deficiency. Vitamin B12 only has animal sources in most cases and supplements are also usually recommended. Although if one is consuming the occasional animal protein, there's usually enough vitamin B12 in one helping of animal protein to last at least a month in terms of supply of vitamin B12 which is very important for prevention of anemia, healthy red blood cells, as well as nerve function.

Adequate iron and calcium intake from plant sources are recommended. You have adequate iron as well as calcium in most vegetables and beans, and these can also be obtained from minimal intake of animal proteins. In the next chapter, we are going to be talking about why your physician does not get you off medications.

CHAPTER TWO

WHY DOES MY PHYSICIAN NOT GET ME OFF MEDS

How much do physicians generally know about alternative routes to disease management?

This generally not taught in medical schools to any significant degree. The portion of the medical curriculum dedicated to the teaching of nutrition is very, very minimal and suboptimal. Everything I personally learnt about nutrition was learnt as a practicing physician. Alternative routes to disease management is not thought to be important to many physicians. This is because it does not follow the traditional pathway of medicine and it is practiced by practitioners who are not generally seen as real "medical doctors". This is a very unfortunate situation.

How much time does it typically take to discuss getting off medications? Well without a system, this can take a really long time because there are lots of dialogue that can ensue if there is no actual system formulated to manage this discussion. However, with a system, time is managed much more efficiently and succinct questions are asked and everything is covered in a matter of minutes. There should be some literature given to the patient to reinforce many of the points made. As we go through easy, simple, and implementable steps, getting patients onto the right path, headed in the right direction. Having lifestyle coach in-house is also very helpful as this individual is able to then further individualize this care of lifestyle changes and good follow-up then ensues with conference calls and shopping trips and cooking classes and things of that nature. Keep things interesting and develop a community sense with the patient.

Does the physician benefit from getting you off medications?

In general, this is perceived as no gain to the physician because there's less need for the patients to follow up with the doctor. In actuality, patients are more likely to see a physician more frequently to prevent disease, as opposed to treat or manage disease. Personally there is more fulfillment in caring for patients that are well than patients that are sick. There will definitely be shorter visits with patients leaving, feeling very accomplished and great about themselves and the physician feeling very fulfilled that they are making a difference, a positive difference in the life of their patient.

Have you been compliant with your doctor's instruction in the past?

The ideal situation would be to show your doctor you will be compliant going forward and you should be able to convince your doctor that you are both on the same page. Let him know that now that you have been placed on a path to wellness, you are more engaged in your care. This tends to be very encouraging to the doctor who generally believes patients are non-compliant. They don't feel it is worth their time to get patients on the right path because they don't stay on it. They tend to generally be very non-compliant. In my experience, sometimes with needed repetition, patients become compliant and actually encourage compliance in their family members.

Does your physician look healthy?

Generally, I suggest to patients to change physicians if they don't want to look the way the physician looks. I would want to buy a suit from an individual dressed in a very sharp suit. I would not be very encouraged to be trained by a trainer who has a pot belly and skinny legs. I suggest to challenge your doc to do what you should be doing to get healthy and monitor his reaction and his willingness to get on the right path himself. You can also ask your doc why he does not resemble what a healthy-looking person should embody. I truly believe all professionals should be held accountable for what they teach and profess. I would not want to have a financial planner who is always broke.

Have you asked for your Medical Doctor to get you off medications?

You should ask your doctor to get you off medications and if he does not know how to do this, then ask him to please research how to get you off medications. Be assertive about the fact that you really want to be off medications by a certain realistic date. Of course, certain medications - especially medications that replace deficient hormones like thyroid medications can't necessarily be stopped but the dose can be optimized by what you eat and your lifestyle.

Have you been bringing in your medications to your doctor visits to discuss?

Bringing in your medications to every doctor's visit becomes very important because as a physician, I am more likely to actively consider getting you off medication when I see the medication in its physical form than I am if I see the medication on a list written by you. You should discuss the need for every medication with your doctor to see if it still needs to be taken. And again discuss what needs to be done to get you off that particular medication. You should ask about the side effects of each medication and then revisit this at each visit.

This marks the end of this chapter.

Asking why your physician doesn't get you off medications? Next chapter, we will be talking about how you can lose weight and keep it off.

CHAPTER THREE

HOW CAN I LOSE WEIGHT AND KEEP IT OFF?

If I exercise twice a day, do I have a better chance at sustained weight loss?

Absolutely, the more exposure you have to exercise, the more calories are consumed. How many days a week should I exercise to keep my weight down? As you get older, you actually need more total exercise.

A perfect example of this is a 20-year-old female requiring 2,100 calories to maintain her weight, but 15 years later required only 1,970 calories to maintain that same weight. If the energy expended does not increase and/or the amount of food taken in does not decrease, those extra 130 calories over a 15 year period will translate to a weight gain of up to 200 pounds. Now, between the age of 35 and age 50 for the same lady, if again she did not increase activity or decrease calorie intake the weight gain may be even more than that. You want to burn more calories than you consume; that is the bottom line. You are more likely to burn more calories if you are giving more time to exercise. I suggest taking one day off per week and when you exercise, pace yourself. Especially in the beginning. Rest as you need to, but show up every time. Preferably twice a day, six days a week. Make a great effort and enjoy it. Stop frequently if you have to but give it the time it deserves.

Am I better doing cardiovascular workouts or weight training?

And does this really result in sustained weight loss? Weight training is important for:

1. Joint position sense.
2. Bone health.
3. Muscle tone amongst other things.

Cardiovascular training is important for:

1. Cardiovascular function.
2. Stamina building.

3. Oxygen utilization.
4. Lung health, also amongst other things.

So as you can see, they both have their advantages and their benefits, and should both be incorporated into your regimen and yes, exercise does result in sustained weight loss. However, it must be consistent and done over time. You must regularly increase how much exercise you do. Start low, as low as five minutes twice a day is sufficient. But then continue to build up to the point where you are doing 30 minutes to an hour, twice a day. Again, have fun doing it. Do exercise that you enjoy doing, which you look forward to doing. But if you don't look forward to doing it, do it anyway. Show up and do it.

Does bariatric surgery result in sustained weight loss?

Well on its own, No. Bariatric surgery is a good modality for patients that are unable to achieve sustained weight loss with non-surgical intervention such as eating habits and exercise. But if bariatric surgery is not complemented with persistent improvement in eating habits and exercise, patient will result in weight loss followed by rebound in weight gain which is actually more dangerous for the patient than if he had not lost the weight in the first place. When body is in starvation mode, because of decreased calorie presented to the gut, as happens in bariatric surgery, the basic metabolic rate goes down. If this is not increased with exercise, the body becomes much more efficient in using less calories. So the body adapts to less calories and stores extra calories presented to it as fat.

What meal is best to cheat with to keep my weight off and prevent weight gain?

If you cheat, cheat with wisdom. It is best to cheat in the morning when cortisol, which is a stress hormone, is highest. This tends to increase metabolic rate and increase energy expenditure. Cheating at night is the worst time to cheat, where cortisol is at its lowest ebb and the metabolic rate is at its lowest. Unless, of course, you increase it with a great workout. When you do cheat, there should be increased exercise and water intake. So again, when you cheat, cheat wisely.

Can I use meds to lose weight and keep it off? Another pill? How do pills work?

In order for pills to result in weight loss, it is obviously blocking a natural process. One could argue that the process it is blocking is deleterious to your health but in most cases, that process being blocked also has some beneficial effects on your health. And so changing your habits so less of the deleterious effects occur, and more of the beneficial effects occur, would be the better way to go. As much as possible, I always suggest to keep things natural. The body we have is amazing, so that we need to get out its way and let it do its thing. I believe foods are much more fun than pills and as Socrates said, let food be thy medicine. Let us go for results and not conveniences of the pill.

How about the Atkins diet?

Ketones results in water loss, so there will be some weight loss as you embark upon a ketogenic diet. But once you introduce sugar again this disappears and the weight creeps back on as the body is rehydrated. Fatty food results in inflammation and chronic inflammation is one of the biggest problems we have in our society today. At least all the affluent diseases found in the first world such as diabetes, hypertension, hyperlipidemia, all resulting in cardiovascular disease, as opposed to the poor diseases found in the third world countries such as parasitic diseases like malaria and diseases resulting from lack of vaccination like polio, or diseases resulting from lack of food like kwashiorkor and malnutrition, marasmus. Or there are vitamin and mineral deficiencies.

What do the studies show about Atkins diet?

Clearly it's been found that a society that has a high intake of animal protein and conversely low intake of fruits and vegetables has a much higher incidence in the rate of cardiovascular disease and death. I do agree with Atkins, however, that the carb portions and content of our food must be reduced.

How about genetics?

When given a gun, it doesn't have to be used. In the same token, you may need to do more than others would need to do because of the genes you have. So it's important that you know you need to exercise more, or you need to eat less fatty food, or you need to eat more vegetables, fruits, and beans, than you would if you didn't have the genes. But do what needs to be done to attain and maintain great health. You can do nothing about the genetics you've been dealt. All you can do is create the environment that gives you optimal health. Environmental factors are much more important than genes. This brings us to the end of this chapter dealing with losing weight and keeping it off.

The next chapter will be discussing how to do with what we can have for breakfast.

CHAPTER FOUR.

WHAT CAN I EAT FOR BREAKFAST?

Have you gotten away from white, refined carbs?

There are several advantages of unrefined carbs. For one, unrefined carbs has a higher fiber content than refined carbs do. The other advantage is that as a result of the higher fiber content, they generally have a lower glycemic index, which is the index that measures the propensity of a carbohydrate to result in an insulin spike.

Other advantages of unrefined carbs have to do with the amount of calories and the caloric density of the carbs which refers to the nutrient to calorie ratio. The disadvantages of refined carbs have to do with the lack of fiber content which results in high glycemic index and higher insulin spikes which, as discussed a little earlier, results in increased fat conversion. Of course, refined carbs also results in more calories being absorbed as a result of lack of fiber and higher calorie density. So this is generally the case when we refine carbs. Realize that when we do partake of refined carbs, we are indulging. As long as indulging is done actively and not passively, we can still be on the right path. The difference between active and passive eating is what I have coined your food conscience. With intention and training you develop a food consciousness and eventually conscience which gives you a big enough "why" to stay on course.

When was the last time you had only fruits?

Berries are the healthiest fruits. You can't have too many fruits, as noted earlier. Studies showed that the only side effect of too many fruits is frequent large, bulky bowel movements. This also goes for patients that have diabetes. As long as you're not taking in animal proteins, which increases the transit time through the gut, resulting in increased absorption of sugar. I actually recommend a fruit fast as a good detoxification regimen, when one has been exposed to too much rich food. Rich food refers to food with a high fat content. Fruits can also be used to make water more interesting. I would suggest chopping up fruits into small bits and putting it into water to give the water some flavor and some chunky bits as you consume your allotted portion of water for the day.

Always think fiber, fruits, veggies, whole wheat grains. You should have more fiber in every meal including breakfast. If there is no fiber in your meal do not consume that meal - make this a policy.

Fibers can be soluble or insoluble and they are both advantageous. Insoluble fibers tend to be able to retain 15 times their weight in water resulting in large bulky stool which is much more easily expelled from the gut. Soluble fiber tends to form a viscous gel that decreases the absorption of empty calories into the bloodstream from the gut. Consuming your vegetables with egg whites makes a great healthy omelet that can be taken with whole wheat bread or sweet potatoes. Oatmeal is an awesome breakfast that you can't go wrong with.

How much time do you give to breakfast?

If planned, breakfast is actually easy. However, if not planned, breakfast tends to be quite unhealthy because then you grab what you can grab quickly and take off. As always, that something is usually going to be something unhealthy except you have enough discipline to grab a fruit on the go. So give time to plan breakfast, know the day before or the night before what you will be having for breakfast. You can actually plan your wake up time such that you have enough time to make the kind of breakfast you want to partake of.

Do you exercise before breakfast?

Having a morning ritual with breakfast being a part of it is something I highly recommend. In this ritual take time to meditate and go through affirmations. Visualize your goals, your desires. Talk to God, pray to Him, fellowship with Him, praise Him, and then exercise. Have a great workout before breakfast. Exercise before any meal including breakfast. It tends to increase the chances of a meal being a healthy meal and drastically decreasing the risk of overeating. A change in motion usually helps and improves your emotion and sets the tone for your day. So I highly recommend a morning ritual inclusive of exercise before your breakfast.

Do you routinely take stimulants in the morning?

Eating foods that stimulates results in the withdrawal phenomenon because stimulation results in the release of feel good hormones which tend to take you on a high. As I said earlier, with the high comes the low and during this low you crave again to be on that high. So the ideal situation is to find an appropriate source of the release of feel good hormones on a regular basis. This usually results in a healthy passion such as exercise or a good relationship with your spouse, your siblings, your children or just a good friend. The best and most reliable source is a great relationship with God. Unfortunately, there are also inappropriate sources of the release of this feel-good hormones, which includes inappropriate sex. So it should be mentioned that sex with your spouse is a fantastic source of the feel-good hormone. But extramarital sex and excessive sex, especially extramarital is not a good source. Intake of rich sweets or fat filled foods is also an inappropriate source. The use of drugs, cigarette smoking, alcohol, even those one that have depressive effects in the brain, all result in the release of this feel-good hormone. Heightened senses occur when you are stealing or doing dangerous things and it also results in the release of this feel-good hormone that are inappropriate sources.

So stimulants taken in the AM to release these feel good hormones are things I discourage because then, the ability to be satisfied with foods that are healthy is much lower as they do not result in the release of these feel-good hormones themselves. That should have been done by the morning ritual before the breakfast and sustained through the day by doing things that you are passionate about, good relationship with work buddies and colleagues. And of course a great relationship with God.

Do you like smoothies?

I recommend smoothies because this is a very convenient way to get your breakfast on the go for those of you that are like me and have many busy mornings. I recommend blending your fruits and not juicing them because that removes the healthy fiber from your smoothie. I suggest adding vegetables to your smoothies and using almond milk as opposed to dairy milk. I recommend adding oatmeal, which has amazing medicinal qualities. I also recommend making large batches of these and freezing them and letting them thaw overnight to be taken on the go as you head out to begin your day.

This brings us to the end of this chapter where we spoke about what you can have for breakfast. Next chapter, we will be discussing which is worse for consumption between simple carbs and fatty food.

CHAPTER FIVE

WHICH IS WORSE FOR ME, SIMPLE CARBS OR FATTY FOODS?

THE THERMOGENIC EFFECT?

This results in energy expenditure that occurs when consumed carbs are converted to fat and stored. Interestingly enough, this results in the expenditure of 25% of the stored energy in fat. This is as opposed to consumed fat being converted to stored fat, in which case only 3% of the stored energy is expended in this conversion. So it is better to convert carbs to fat than converting fat to fat. This means the healthier of the two evils in this situation would be the carbs.

Of course, I am referring to the simple carbs. There are less calories per gram in carbs than in fat - four calories per gram of carbs, while there are nine calories per gram of fat.

Simple vs complex carbs - Packaging

So simple carbs should be preferred over fatty foods but preferably complex carbs should be taken. Complex carbs have a depot effect, with a decreased insulin spike. This results from the fiber content of these complex carbs with all the great benefits that have already been listed for great fiber content. You can make your choice instantaneously healthier by adding fiber for improved packaging. Packaging is a term I give to what is presented to the gut when we eat. Food ideally should be packaged with fiber so that the gut more easily transports the package through it and expels it with as little absorption into the blood as possible. This is much better with fiber than without. If you are going to indulge, indulge with wisdom

Whether this is fatty foods or simple carbs, do it with wisdom. This should be when:

- The basal metabolic rate is highest, which tends to be in the morning.
- You are less likely to be sedentary
- We use the ability to detoxify the body with fruits, vegetable and water taken with small portions of the carbs.
- Let inflammation subside

- Give time for inflammation, which is triggered by the fatty food, to subside before the next insult with this fatty food.

This is why I recommend for fatty food to be taken much less frequently and the frequency of the intake of fatty food is much more important that the quantity of fatty food taken because the inflammation that is triggered by the fatty food will peak and then subside if there is no more exposure of the fatty food to the lining of the blood vessels. However, if this exposure is done continuously, then inflammation becomes a chronic problem as the lining of the blood vessels now work like a pharmacy gone crazy just dispensing drugs without any prescriptions.

See them for what they are -indulgences

Indulgences are indulgences whether we are referring to fatty food or simple carbs. So enjoy the indulgence knowing that that is exactly what it is - an indulgence. Knowing that this is an indulgence should make consuming them fewer and far between. Indulge as a reward for achieving milestones or reaching your goals or various things you can think of to reward yourself for.

Do not reward yourself too often, actively plan for them. Plan ahead of time for these indulgences and make an effort to be more, even more able to withstand the effects of the indulgences by what you do leading up to the planned day. This means more exercise, more water intake, more fruits, vegetables, beans, rest.

Avoid having these foods around the house, be it fatty foods or simple carbs. When you consume them, consume them as part of a celebration outside your home. Agree with others at home to have these consumed outside and not at home. Agree with everyone at home to avoid keeping them in the house and constantly plan to have these indulgences outside at specific times.

Eat with an awareness

Make sure your eating or partaking of these indulgences is done with an active as opposed to a passive attitude. This means you are aware of what you are consuming and you are not just mindlessly consuming. Chances are higher of active consumption if they are consumed slowly. Chances of this being the case is also higher if they are consumed with less distraction, that is, not consuming while watching the game or watching a movie but sitting down without the distractions and eating slowly.

Calories are much higher in fatty food

Calories are much higher in fatty food just by way of the caloric density, ie. the amount of calories per unit of volume. This is much higher with fatty food. The nutrient to calorie ratio is also important. The nutrient portion of the food can be increased by taking low calorie density foods alongside options such as fruits and vegetables.

This brings us to the end of this chapter, dealing with the question of which one being worse between the consumption of simple carbs or fatty foods. In the next chapter we shall be dealing with "Is eating fish healthy?".

CHAPTER SIX

IS EATING FISH HEALTHY?

Fish contains healthy fats, but more importantly also contains unhealthy fats. Fish contains omega three fatty acids, which make up some of the essential fatty acids and these are important for various things. However, fat calories are still calories and there are more calories in fat than there are in carbs. Fish contains no fiber whatsoever and unhealthy fats are a strong initiator of inflammation.

Countries or cultures that eat fish have been found to have more disease. Certain cultures where intake of fish is prevalent, chronic disease is generally much more prevalent. These were found in the China study which was a landmark study showing these associations. In this same culture, there is more evident bone disease as a result of the increased acidity of the blood resulting from the fish which leads to increased calcium being leached from the bones into the blood. This results in hypercalcemia i.e. high calcium content in the blood which leads to high calcium in urine and the formation of kidney stones and of course osteoporosis. There is also more cardiovascular disease in these patients as a result of fish.

Eating food with no fiber leads to constipation

Generally, fiber forms a skeleton for the easier packaging that I alluded to earlier which results in the formation of large bulky stools which are more easily expelled. Of course fiber causes a decrease in transit time, resulting in less absorption of calories, as the food transits through the gut much quicker. Which is not the case with fish. Without fiber, walls of the gut continue to slip over the food as the wall is unable to achieve traction. This is as opposed to good traction propelling food forward, which happens mostly with food that contain fiber.

Kidney stone formation

Fatty food/animal proteins create an acidic pH in the blood and this results in more stone formation. There is literature about animal proteins in general, including fish resulting in a more acidic medium which results in more stone formation. The opposite applies with fruits and vegetables which result in a more alkaline medium which causes the calcium to be retained by the bone and decreases the incidence of kidney stones.

Kidney stones, incidentally, causes pain which has been described as nearest experience for a man to come to experiencing childbirth or the nearest situation a man can go through to experiencing pain of childbirth.

Fat calories are more than carb calories

Calories are calories and if not burned, they are stored as fat. Stored fat in the wrong place leads to inflammation and Inflammation in return, leads to the formation of an unstable plaque which increases the risk of cardiovascular events and also leads to the formation of cancerous cells. It also leads to alteration of DNA with the formation of autoimmune disorders.

As a general rule, do not consume more than you can burn. Aim to consume less calories than you will burn. As mentioned above, thermogenesis occurs when fats or carbs are converted to the stored form of fuel which is fat. 25% of energy being stored is used up in the case of carbs being converted to fat while only 3% is used up when consumed fat is converted to body fat, so consume carbs over fats.

Fatty tissue is a very large store of toxins. Most toxins are consumed orally in food or inspired air or through the skin and are typically stored in fat. Fat consumed is also medium for toxins to get into our system. Detoxification is discouraged by excessive fatty stores.

Unhealthy fat is a key ingredient for inflammation. Again, inflammation refers to the various signs that result from injury to any part of the body, as evidenced by swelling, redness, heat, and pain. This is the acute response to injury, that is acute inflammation. This will eventually subside as the various cells that are recruited result in reversal of the damage done. The problem is when this becomes a chronic problem and maladaptive responses occur that lead to the chronic diseases that plague our society today. The most common causes of death making up almost 80-85% of all deaths in America result from inflammation, chronic inflammation. These include cardiovascular disease, cancers, strokes and chronic obstructive pulmonary disease. The biggest trigger of inflammation is unhealthy fat. Of course the effects of chronic inflammation are the biggest drivers for these prescription medications today.

This brings us to the end of this chapter, dealing with is eating fish healthy? In the next chapter we will be dealing more with how much sleep one really needs per night?

CHAPTER SEVEN

HOW MUCH SLEEP DO I REALLY NEED PER NIGHT?

Do you typically feel sleepy during the day?

Alertness through the day dictates if sleep is enough. Also the need for frequent catnaps are also an indication as to whether you are getting enough sleep or not. Headaches will also be another indicator. Frequent headaches through the day are a very common sin of a sleep deprivation. Also, sleepiness through the day could also be evidence of the presence of the obstructive sleep apnea syndrome or one the other causes of fragmented sleep.

How much sleep have you had on average, over the last month?

What is the average number of hours of sleep per night you have had over the last month. Do you feel optimal through the day? This will be an indicator as to whether you are having your optimal amount of sleep. Do you wake up feeling refreshed, which is also very important or do you hit the snooze button several times before you wake up. Are there any signs of chronic sleep deprivation such as bags under your eyes or bloodshot eyes?

Are you overweight? Are you having weight gain or weight loss? How many hours of sleep do you get before midnight. In general, every hour of sleep before midnight is an equivalent to one and a half hours of sleep after midnight.

Obesity becomes a problem as a result of the hormonal imbalance that results from fragmented sleep, when there's an increase in the number of awake hormones in ratio to the number of sleep hormones, which results in weight gain and difficulty sustaining weight loss.

Do you have trouble falling asleep?

Trouble falling asleep will trigger certain questions to be asked such as, is there a TV in the bedroom? This has been found to be a very important factor in preventing people from falling asleep, unbeknownst to them. Are you depressed? If you are suffering from depression, one of the signs of this is difficulty in falling asleep. And sometimes until this is treated, this remains a highly prominent symptom of depression. Avoid eating three hours before bedtime. This can affect your ability to sleep.

Does everyone need eight hours of sleep?

Not everyone needs eight hours of sleep. Some people thrive on much less sleep than that, so it is obvious that the amount of sleep actually required is very individualized. It is more important to plan to be up at a predetermined time before sleeping. Although studies have shown that most people need between six to eight hours of sleep a day, some people do thrive on less hours of sleep per day. This needs to be individualized, making sure the signs of sleep deprivation or fragmented sleep direct you as to how much sleep you should actually be having per night.

The body's defense system is more optimal with adequate sleep. The body's defense system is referred to as the immune system and it is indeed enhanced by adequate rest. This is evidenced by improved wound healing and ability to better weather viral illnesses as they occur when there is adequate sleep. The immune system is definitely depressed by fatigue and increased stress results from inadequate sleep. This leads on its own to a myriad of symptoms, including a depressed immune system. You are more likely to develop symptoms of a viral illness when you are sleep deprived as opposed to someone with adequate sleep if both of you are exposed to the same virus.

Risk of diabetes increases with lack of sleep

Risk of diabetes increases with lack of sleep. This is also the case with obesity. And this results again from the ratio of awake hormones to the ratio of sleep hormones reversing which results in glucose intolerance which leads over time to diabetes.

Fragmented sleep actually results in the release of these awake hormones as opposed to being at a lower level during sleep. With the increased amount of these awake hormones which are also stress hormones as well as adrenaline, there's an increase in the glucose intolerance which leads to diabetes.

THE ENDING CHAPTER

We have been able to go through a chapters dealing with how we can get off prescription medications. Followed by a chapter dealing with why your physician does not get you off medications. And then we delved into how you can lose weight and keep it off. Followed by what you can have for breakfast. Then we debated on which was worse for you between simple carbs and fatty food. Then we pondered whether eating fish is healthy. And finally discussed how much sleep you will need per night.

Take action to achieve not having to worry about taking medications every day, being in good health, and being filled with pride every time the doctor says you are doing great. The first step is to call my office at **407-297-8408** asking to speak to Stephanie and tell her I want to take advantage of Dr. Awosika's ultimate 21 day plant based detox and she will get you all set up.

www.ingramcontent.com/pod-product-compliance
Lightning Source LLC
Chambersburg PA
CBHW070305190526
45169CB00004B/1527